Does Nora Five-element Acupuncture Depend mostly on Psychological Effect?

Dr. Martin Wang MD. PhD

Edmonton, Canada[1]

Abstract: Five-element theory was developed in acupuncture in China. It was then passed to Japan, Korea and then to the UK. After that, its concept and its application in the diagnosis and treatment of diseases have been changed dramatically. The UK's Five-element acupuncture system (hereafter known as Nora Five-element acupuncture) depends on a patient's life story, voice, skin color and the smell/odor of the body in setting up a diagnosis for the dominant element of the body (e.g. one of the five elements: Wood, Fire, Soil, Metal and Water).

In treatment, the method emphasizes the personal relationship between the acupuncturist and the patient. The acupuncture is used as a complementary means of treatment and is used mostly to nourish the dominant element of the body, and to conduct the meridian energy from other meridians to the dominant element meridian, not caring for the various relationships among the elements (such as nourishing, restraining, reverse restraining, etc.).

Before a typical Five-element acupuncture treatment, some other clinical conditions have to be treated first, such as Attached body, Aggressive body energy, Blockage of energy

[1] Wenqiw57@hotmail.com

flow between meridians, Unbalanced pulse (Left-right unbalance), scar tissue blockage, etc. The diagnosis and treatment of these conditions mostly has nothing to do with the Five-element theory. Therefore, we predict that the diagnosis of this acupuncture system is difficult to be accurate. It requires a very high personal ability from the acupuncturist (communication skills, the sense of body language, skin color and body odor, the willingness to come into patient's emotional life, etc.). The placebo effect might take large part of the whole healing effect. The so-called Five-element is only a small part of the whole acupuncture treatment. Furthermore, the treatment of various disease conditions, and the improvement of the symptoms after the treatment, could enhance the placebo effect and also tend to let the acupuncturist believe that the previous diagnosis of body-dominated element is correct.

During the so-called Five-element acupuncture course, the choice of many acupuncture points is not related to the Five-element theory. This acupuncture system is recommended mostly for the treatment of emotionally oriented issues, not for physically oriented or "out-oriented" diseases, so the favorite disease spectrum is narrow. Because there are so many differences between this UK Five-element acupuncture and the Traditional Five-element system in China, we recommend the launch of a clinical comparison study, to see if such modified acupuncture techniques could really contribute to the treatment of emotional issues, with or without the strongly recommended, very good personal relationship between acupuncturist and the patient, and with or without care of the mutual nourish-restrain relationship between the elements.

Contents

Introduction:

《Five element acupuncture》 [1] is a book written by Nora Flaglen. It was recently translated by acupuncturist Long Mei into Chinese. Here we discuss the Chinese version of the book. This book gained some interest in China. A Traditional Chinese Medicine scholar named Liu Li-hong praised it. The author said that the Five-element acupuncture technique originated in China, passed to Japan, then Korea and then later to the UK. What's unique about the UK's Five-element acupuncture is that it separates people into five elements, finds the dominant element of the patient, and uses acupuncture to nourish the dominant element to bring balance to the five elements in the body.

After reading the book, we found that the Nora Five-element theory used in the UK's Five-element acupuncture system is largely different from traditional Five-element theory in China. It is not easy to learn, the parameters for diagnosis of the dominant element of the body's constitution is not clear enough, it takes a long time for improvement, the improvement appears slowly, and the healing effect is hard to predict. We feel that it is necessary to make a comparison study to compare Nora Five-element acupuncture with traditional acupuncture, especially with Pan's Yin-Yang acupuncture system, to see if the former, with its modified Five-element theory, would really work better than other acupuncture systems.

1   Main characteristics of Nora Five-element acupuncture

The Nora Five-element acupuncture system aims to find the dominant element of the body's constitution. The dominant body element is believed to be one of the five elements: Wood, Fire, Soil [2], Metal and Water. It is believed that a disease, especially an emotional problem of the body, is due to weakness of the dominant element. The aim of the treatment is to nourish the weakened dominant element, so as to bring the dominant element up to normal levels.

---

[2] Most of books use the word "Earth" here. We feel that this is not the proper word for the translation. The word 'earth' is the name of a planet, parallel to the names of other planets, such as sun, Mars, Saturn, or Mercury. The word 'Soil' here is more close to its meaning: butter, transformer, lubricate.

1.1 Diagnosis

The author, Nora Fleglan, admitted that the constitution of the body could have a mixed pattern, if it is diagnosed according to the Five-element theory. However, everyone must have his or her own one dominant element. The acupuncturist needs to find the dominant element. Each of the five elements has various differences. The author paid most attention to the personality, the way of speaking, the voice, the skin color and the body odor, to separate the five elements and to find out the dominant element for each patient.

Using the acupuncture point temperature test (Akabane Test), the pulse diagnosis, and abdomen touch diagnosis, the author admitted that the pulse diagnosis is the most accurate method of diagnosis, but she did not use it for the diagnosis of the body's dominant element. The acupuncture point temperature test could find out the imbalance of life energy flow between meridians, but the information obtained by this method was not used to find the body's dominant element either. It seems that none of these ways of diagnosis were used for the diagnosis of the body's dominant element.

During diagnosis, it is best for the acupuncturist to quickly feel the dominated body element of the patient using instinct and emotion. It is not recommended that the acupuncturist analyses the information collected. It is better to use non-logical feelings rather than the logical analysis of the mind.

1.2 Treatment

Even after diagnosis is set up, treatment for the dominant element cannot start until pre-existing conditions are dealt with first: "Attached spirit", "Aggressive energy", energy flow blockage, imbalanced left-right pulse, scar tissue blockage, etc. (Hereafter we name all of these conditions as pre-treatment conditions.). The diagnosis and the treatment for these pre-treatment conditions basically have nothing to do with Five-element theory.

In Five-element treatment, the aim is to nourish the Qi and Blood in the dominant element, with the belief that emotional disorders are due to the weakness of the dominant element, though it has been mentioned that we can use depletion technique acupuncture in cases where the dominant element is overwhelming.

Using depletion with Five-element theory means depleting the following element (the son element), if the given element is in overwhelming (excess) condition, or to nourish the previous element (the mother element), if the given element is weak (deficient) condition, e.g. the Mother-son principle. However, Nora also uses the principle to deplete and to nourish the same element the same time. The technique also uses the depletion or nourishment of grandmother or grandson. The latter two methods are rare in traditional Chinese Five-element theory.

Before using Five-element acupuncture, the Nora method uses moxibustion first to stimulate the acupuncture points, then uses acupuncture needles for stimulation. We insert a needle on the left side of the body first for nourishing technique, or on the right side first for depletion technique. For the depletion technique, we leave the needle in the acupuncture point for about 20 minutes, and for the nourishing technique, the needle is taken out right away after the Deqi sensation is felt (no retention of the needle). We apply the direction of the needle along or against the direction of energy flow in the meridians to reach the nourishment or depletion effect.

After Nora Five-element acupuncture is performed, the method always uses needles to stimulate the Primary point of the meridians. We may also stimulate the points according to the season. For example, if it is Spring (Spring belongs to Wood), the acupuncture points in the Liver and Gall bladder meridian (Both meridians also belong to Wood) might be also stimulated.

Acupuncture is performed once a week in most cases, for 6 to 8 total sessions.

1.3   Healing Results

With diagnosis and treatment, the acupuncturist needs to evaluate and to access the healing effect of previous treatments every time, to see if the previous diagnosis of the dominant element is correct. Even after 6-8 weeks (6-8 sessions) of treatment, it is hard to know if the element diagnosis is correct or not.

Whether the element diagnosis is correct or not depends on the improvement of physical symptoms, as well as if the patient becomes happier emotionally, or more willing to talk, etc.

1.4   Dominant pattern of diseases

As introduced in the book, the dominant diseases that are better treated with this style of acupuncture are the inner-oriented diseases, e.g. those diseases which are caused by emotional imbalance/disorder, such as anger, depression, frustration, fear, loneliness, etc., not for ordinary out-oriented diseases, such as Wind, Cold, Hot, Wetness, Dryness, Fire, Water, etc. It is also not used for physical trauma, such as falling down, bruises, of being bitten by animals or insects.

2   Analysis of the Nora Five-element acupuncture system

2.1   Diagnosis

The author makes the Five-element diagnosis of the body's dominant element based on the study of personality, voice, skin color, and body odor. The author admits that it is very difficult to make the diagnosis: "For many years, I have gradually set up my own way of the diagnosis, but in practice, there were mistakes again and again. The clue for a given element in a patient seems quite opposite the characteristics that I have set up in my mind before. It might be because my understanding of the characteristics of that element is immature. Therefore I have to always remind myself: it seems impossible to separate people according to the five elements. In reality, everyone can show various mild differences from others." (p14)[3]

"The diagnosis of the five elements is a long time of courses in which it is needed to filter the sensations of us towards the patients. It is needed to

---

[3] The number in parentheses is the page number in the Chinese translated version of book *Guide of Five-element Acupuncture* (reference 1).

isolate the various different signals emitted by the five elements, and to identify the most dominated one. This needs our ability and patience. It is a very long time to spend." (p49)

"It is very complex the five element diagnosis. It asks us to spend long time to filter the signals from organs and from other sources." (p88)

If the developer of Nora Five-element acupuncture feels so confused, how about others who learn this technique?

For various information collected from patient, the highest level of diagnosis is a fast telepathy, not the analytical results from the mind of the acupuncturist. Therefore, different acupuncturists will have different evaluation results of the patient's emotional and personal status. If we ask the acupuncturist why he or she made one diagnosis but not another, he or she might answer, I just feel that it should be this one (no reason given).

Different patients have different diseases or problems to solve. Generally speaking, when a patient comes to an acupuncturist, the patient wants to solve the current problem that the patient feels bothers him or her too much. Therefore, the patient does not want the doctor to shift the treatment goal to something else that the patient does not feel is urgent to solve, and the patient is hesitant to answer questions that the patient feels are not directly related to the current problem. This is very common in acupuncture clinics. If a patient suffers from cough, and if we ask the patient how about his or her bowel movement, the patient feels strange about why we ask such questions, so they tend to not to answer with the truth. Only after we have solved the problem that the patient feels is most urgent, then they start to ask if we can continue to help him or her with some other problems.

For example, a patient comes the first time to see if we can reduce the pain in his lower back. If we asked him what about his sleeping, he might say that it is not bad or not too bad. After the lower back pain subsides, the patient then asks if we are also able to improve his sleep, because he has been taking sleeping pill for many years. This example means that it is not easy to get the truth from patients in the initial sessions of treatment and it is not easy to advance into the life of a patient before the patient experiences success from the treatments.

According to the Five-element theory, Wood and Fire persons tend to be extroverted, Metal and Water persons tend to be introverted, and Soil persons are general. This means that Metal and Water persons are hesitant to answer questions, especially if the question is related to private life. The acupuncturist is not always lucky in getting answer from all of his clients. In clinics, some patients tend to talk a lot, and others are very silent and only answer questions when you ask them.

The reliability of patient body odor as diagnostic evidence is not high. In Western countries, many patients come to the clinic after having showered. The body odor is not clear. Patients from other countries tend to come after they eat, so the body is rich from curry. Also some people like to use a lot of Western herbal lotions, or perfume, or something for bromhidrosis. The odor is too strong and can create a headache for the acupuncturist.

It is the same for skin color. In Western countries, it is easy to meet people with dark or brown skin color. It is meaningless to see their skin color for element diagnosis. We might only be able to check their mucus color in mouth, palm or eye lid. However, if the mucus color changes in these places to suggest a diagnosis, the condition is already very severe and the patient should go to hospital, not to an acupuncture clinic. Once a patient uses lipstick, we cannot see the true color in the lip either. Also, if a disease is new, the skin color would not change dramatically.

In the article, it said that we need to check the color and tint of the skin. Probably only an acupuncturist with very accurate sense of color could sense the difference of color tint among some patients.

The commonly used methods of diagnosis in Traditional Chinese Medicine, such as pulse diagnosis, tongue diagnosis, and palpation diagnosis, are not applied here for the diagnosis of the dominant element of the body's constitution. This means that the author does not believe that the information collected by these traditional ways would have anything related to body element constitution. However, in the chapter on treatment, the author said, "if the pulse diagnosis suggests the Qi deficiency in the meridian, use nourish technique (p110)." and "If the pulse suggests the excess of Qi in the meridian, use depletion technique (p111)." It might be that, the opinion of the author that, if any meridian shows excess evidenced by the pulse, then use depletion technique, and if any meridian shows deficiency evidenced by the pulse, use nourish technique. From the whole book, it seems that the author did not relate the Five-element information from the pulse diagnosis to the access of body element constitution.

In reality, the results of pulse diagnosis, tongue diagnosis and palpitation diagnosis are variable among TCM doctors. The results of body element diagnosis using information from patient's emotional behavior, speaking voice, skin color, body order, are much more variable. This is another reason that it is not easy to get a correct body element diagnosis with the Nora acupuncture system.

According to the book, an acupuncturist should have vision as sharp as an eagle, smell as sharp as a hunting dog, hearing ability as sharp as a fox, intuition as sharp as an infant, as well as compassion as great as Buda's. Anyone with one such ability would be regarded as a superman. How can anyone have all of them? If no such super ability exists, the acupuncturist must practice again and again. This means that the time needed to reach such high super ability might be much more than several years. So, before the acupuncturist gains such super ability, his or her diagnosis is hardly accurate.

The author also admits that the body element constitution could be a mixture of more than two elements, yet wants to find the dominant element. The question is: how do we tell which is the dominant element? If body constitution is 50% Wood, 30% Soil, and 20% Fire, it would be hard to tell if the body constitution is actually Wood or Fire, because the body constitution could be affected by various factors, such as seasons, family life, job environment, relationships, etc. The Wood element might be stronger than Fire in summer, or the Fire element might be stronger than Soil in later summer.

The season in which the emotional condition becomes improved or worse can be used to suggest body element. A Wood constitution might get worse emotionally in fall (Metal), because the Metal counteracts and restrains the Wood. But the emotion of the Wood person could become worse just because the Wood person meets a Metal boss!

If the diagnosis is not for sure, the treatment would be easy to get wrong.

Additionally, the acupuncturist also has his or her own body element. If the dominated element is Wood, or Fire (such as the author herself), or Soil, the acupuncturist may be willing to meet people and talk with people. But if his body element is Metal or Water, he may be hesitant to come into another's personal emotional world. Theoretically, Metal is cooler, strict, and introvert personality and Water is shy and not good at expressing himself. To ask many questions from patients, to come deep into another's life, is a big challenge for them. If the acupuncturist asks many personal questions from the patients, would the patients also be able to ask questions about the acupuncturist himself?[2] If so, the accuracy of personal information collected by such shy acupuncturists is in doubt. This means that about 2/5 of patients and 2/5 of acupuncturists might not be suitable to try such an emotion-related acupuncture treatment.

The author admits too that, during the writing of the book and in the chapter about Wood, she herself felt uneasy emotionally: "I found myself want to escape from the Wood, for its contrast sharply with tit for tat. It is the requirement of the Wood to me. It makes me feel pressure...... I have also to admit that my experience with my family also affect my view of the Wood, some are positive and some negative. Therefore I cannot evaluate the Wood in a very positive way. It always stirs out some irritation from my heart." (p15)

Apparently, acupuncturists can have different feelings for different patients. For some, they like to stay together, for others, they do not. After coming into a patient's personal life, the acupuncturist may find that he may not agree with the patient about some behavior, attitude or way of thinking. Sometimes the acupuncturist may strongly disagree with the patient on the way of dealing with their personal life. As an ordinary person, an acupuncturist might be able to choose to stop a personal relationship with a patient, but as an acupuncturist, he or she has to continue to deal with the patient with a peaceful, neutral, and sympathetic heart. What a big challenge for the acupuncturist!

Without compassion as great as Buda's and without freedom to comment on a patient's behavior, it is hard to prevent positive or negative feelings for the patient. Among current acupuncture systems that we can examine[3], no any other acupuncture system creates such stress for an acupuncturist.

The author herself belongs to Fire element. This is the element that is suitable for walking into another's life (p16), because Fire people are "extremely kind, general, and open" and have "open arms to hold the world", and they "influence the people around him, as the sunshine shines over everything".

Furthermore, there are the Five elements for disease as well. In diagnosis, the author seems to have paid much attention to the body constitution element, but not to the element nature of a disease. But in treatment, the attention is paid more to the Five-element nature of a disease. The Five elements of a body constitution may not necessarily be the same as that of a disease. For example, if a Wood person suffers from cough and diarrhea or asthma (the cough, diarrhea, and asthma can be related to Lung or Large intestine in Chinese medicine, all belonging to Metal), should we treat him as Wood, or as Metal? It is not clearly discussed in the book.

In the book, whenever there are examples for treatment, the element nature of the body constitution and the disease are the same. It is easy to induce the element nature of the disease. For example, in the book, a Wood patient suffered from digestive disease (because the Liver Wood restrains and compresses Soil – the digestive system belongs to Soil) (p18). A Soil patient suffered from swelling in ankles (Spleen Soil fails to restrain the Kidney, the Water), and stomach spasms (Stomach belongs to Soil too. This is the disease of Soil) (p29). A Water patient suffered from severe lower back pain (the lower back houses the Kidney, the Water organ. This is a disease of the Water) (p40).

2.2   Treatment

The book emphasized very much the personal relationship between the acupuncturist and the patient: "Only the warm created from mutual communication between the acupuncturist and the patient could improve the progress of the treatment. Without this, nothing can be obtained with the diagnosis and treatment." (p47)

"It should be kept in mind that, if the treatment is not restricted for physical disease, the highest level of therapy, if it can be said so, is the relationship between the acupuncturist and the patient. Therefore, we should develop a therapy, asking ourselves to be able to create a good environment, to make the patient feel comfort and safe." (p108)

This means that, if an acupuncturist feels unskilled at developing a good relationship with his patient (not everyone in the world has such good skill), then he or she would not be able to expect good healing results in the use of this kind of acupuncture.

However, the author also said, "… even for some acupuncture points which seems not attractive can conduct and contact with the most inner side of the body and the life, and the influence from the deep core will pass to the whole body." (p54) So, if any acupuncture point can reach the deep corners of the body and influence the treatment, why, without a good relationship, can good treatment results not be expected?

But the author again said, "Do not think that the success of the treatment is due to the use of a given or a specific acupuncture point – this is common mistake. The success is the results of our efforts to enhance the structural balance of the five elements. The treatment is a gradual course…." (p81) So, is the success due to the efforts to enhance the structural balance of the five elements, not in solely depending on the "good relationship" between the acupuncturist and patient?

To spend two hours in the first acupuncture session is very difficult in China, especially in bigger hospitals where every doctor has to see more than 40, 60, or 80 patients per day, everyday. In a clinic, we always keep a neutral mind/heart to see every patient. We try to improve the symptoms of the patients and then gain the trust of patients in order to set up the confidence of patients and continue the treatment. Without any improvement each time, patients would not return. After the establishment of trust with patients for the improvement of the diseases that they want to solve, we can start to talk more about the reasons for their stress, frustration, anxiety or depression. At this state, patients are ready to listen to us.

The slow process that the author created can only be used in a clinic that is not busy and we have to charge more for each patient for the survival of the clinic. We know that it is better to have a good relationship with patients and take care of them more from the emotional aspect, but in current medical systems, both Western and Chinese, e have to take care a large number of clients every day; a deep and good relationship between an acupuncture and patients is a dream. We have to take a certain number of clients every day so that we can keep the cost of the treatment reasonable, at a point which most clients can afford.

The Nora Five-element acupuncture system requires a sequence of treatments: if there are some special disease conditions, such as "Attached spirit", "Aggressive energy", blockage of life energy flow in meridians, imbalance of left-right pulse, scar tissue, these pre-treatment conditions should be treated before the typical Five-element acupuncture. This suggests that the Five-element therapy here is basically not so capable of solving such pre-treatment conditions. It is therefore a limited therapy for some kinds of diseases but not for these pre-treatment conditions.

It can be expected that, after the above pre-treatment conditions are corrected, if the pre-treatment indeed works, the body condition, as well as the emotional condition of a patient, should also be improved at the same time. It would be strange if the improvement of a physical disease is not accompanied by the improvement of the emotional disorder. Therefore, we strongly believe that the treatment of these conditions have already improved the emotional status of the patients, before the application of later typical Five-element acupuncture. It is quite common in our daily clinic that with the improvement of physical diseases from acupuncture treatment, patients become much more peaceful and calm.

2.2.1   "Attached spirit"

Diagnosis: Look straight into the eye of the patient. If there is "Attached spirit", the patient will feel constrained and uneasy upon receiving the stare.

Treatment: Inner Seven-needle acupuncture therapy or outer Seven-needle acupuncture therapy. The application of these acupuncture techniques has nothing to do with the Five-element theory.

2.2.2   "Aggressive energy" (AE)

Diagnosis: In the following conditions, there may be AE in the body: if the patient shows irritation; if the patient cries easily; if there is pain in the chest or upper back; if there is muscle tightness on the back; if there is a skin rash on the back; if there is white colored skin at the spot of needle; if there is a rash on the skin around the needle.

Treatment: Every patient needs to have the treatment for expelling the AE in the first session. Acupuncture is done on the back Shu points (both sides beside the spine). If the AE remains and is not being expelled, continue the treatment in following sessions. Without clearing the AE, any following treatment will be to no avail.

The author said, "if there is the AE, the skin rash around the needle continues and not disappear with time (if there is a comparison needle beside, the skin rash will subside with time). Keep the needle until the skin rash subsides (e.g. until the AE depletes off the body)." "Even if the AE has been expelled out of the body, there is still slight rash for additional 10-15 minutes around the needle hole, it might be due to the skin reaction to the needle. It still means that the AE has been expelled off." (p146) "If the skin rash does not subside along the time, it means there is no AE".

It seems that with or without AE, there could be a skin rash around the needle. The skin rash due to the AE will or will not subside with time? It is confusing.

The author said, "the sequence of the passing of the AE follows the restraint sequence of the five elements. It only passes from solid organ to solid organ (e.g. from Kidney Water – Spleen Soil- Liver Wood – Lung Metal- to Heart Fire), not from hollow organ to hollow organ (e.g. not among the Small intestine, Large intestine, Gall bladder, Urine bladder, and Stomach). So, why can't the presence of the AE be evidenced in pulse diagnosis so as to only treat the organ and its corresponding Back Shu point on the body back, rather than stimulating all the Back Shu? According to the author, it seems that the pulse diagnosis cannot help in this regard, so all the Back Shu points have to be stimulated with needles.

Our own experience is that it is very common to have a skin rash around acupuncture needles on the back. The skin rash can be bigger or smaller. The patient with such a skin rash will improve much faster than those without a skin rash or with very little skin rash. There could be allergic reaction to needles. In this case, the skin rash could be dark red in color; the patient usually will feel a strong itch or even pain and the needle is tightly adhered to the skin. However, an allergic reaction to acupuncture needles is very rare. Surely we can also regard the allergic reaction to needle as a kind of AE.

2.2.3   Imbalance of left-right pulse

Diagnosis: The left pulse is weak but the right pulse is strong. Or, more specifically, the Heart pulse on the left side of wrist is weak. Or the pulse on the three positions on the right wrist is surprisingly stronger and the patients shows as hopeless.

Treatment: Conduct the energy from meridians on the right side to those on the left side.

In the treatment, it is necessary to nourish the Heart, the Liver and the Kidney meridians, since the Qi-Blood status of all the three organs are reflected on the pulse on the left wrist.

In the treatment, it is necessary to nourish the Zhiyin (BL67) point (the Metal point on the Urine bladder meridian) on the left side. Metal nourishes the Water.

Nourish the Taixi (KD3) point (the Soil point on the Kidney meridian). The Soil restrains the Water, though it is the Primary point of the Urine bladder meridian. We suggest stimulating the Water point on the Water meridian, the Yingu (KD10) point (Water point).

Nourish the Zhongfeng (LV4) point (Metal point) on the Liver meridian (Wood). The Metal restrains the Wood. It is the brake point on the Liver meridian.

It is also necessary to stimulate the Primary point on the Small intestine meridian (Fire), the Wangu (GB12). It is better to stimulate the Qiangu (SI2) point (Water point, the brake point) in the Small intestine meridian, so as to reduce the Qi flow (descending) in the Small intestine meridian and to indirectly help the Heart Meridian (to ascend).

2.2.4   Blockage for the energy flow in meridians

There could be some blockage of the life energy flow from meridian to meridian. It can only be diagnosed with pulse diagnosis. It might also show as changes in color, voice, or some emotional aspect, or some physical sign around the blocked area of the body. For example, for a blockage between Wood and Metal, this would show as a relatively stronger pulse in the Liver position, while the pulse on the Lung position was relatively weaker. This is called Liver-Lung blockage. The pulse shows the Liver pulse is tight but that the Lung pulse is somehow hollow-like. There could be some other signs to suggest the blockage, such as being easily irritated, tightness or pain in the chest, or pale face (the sign of disorder in the Liver or Lung meridian).

Treatment: Take the Liver/Lung blockage as example: Nourish the outlet of the Liver meridian: Qimen (LV14) point (both sides, first left, then right side); Nourish the inlet of the Lung meridian: the Zhongfu (LU1) point (both sides, also left first).

2.2.5   Blockage due to scar tissue

This means that the energy flow is blocked by scar tissue, caused by surgical operation or trauma.

Treatment: Insert needle above and below the scar tissue. Use nourish technique.

2.2.6   Five-element treatment

After solving the various pre-treatment disorders above, and if the patient still feels discomfort or disorders, Nora Five-element treatment starts.

The author admits that, "For any element, the energy flow is too much or too little in it would hurt health." (p51)

However, the author still paid much attention in the treatment of the dominant element of the body when it is in a weakened condition. So, the treatment principle is to nourish the dominant Element, because, "One of the most principle in the Five-element therapy for most cases is the nourish circle of the five elements." (p96) This means that the author believes that the disease of an Element is due to weakness of the Element, and she does not care if associated emotional disorders are caused by overwhelming of the dominant element of the body. When the author tells us about the characteristics of each Element, she mostly talks about the manifestation of Element deficiency, not that of Element overwhelming.

For treatment, nourish the mother acupuncture point in the given meridian, do not use the mother point in the mother meridian. For example, if the dominant Soil is weak, nourish the Jiexi (ST41) point (the Fire point in the Stomach (Soil) meridian) and nourish the Dadu (SP2) point (the Fire point in the Spleen (Soil) meridian). The book does not mention nourishing the Shaofu (ST8) point (Fire point in the Heart (Fire) meridian), or Yanggu (SI5) point (Fire point in the Small intestine (Fire) meridian), Laogong (PC8) (Fire point in the Heart shell (Fire) meridian), or Zhigou (TH6) (Fire point in the Triple Jiao (Fire) meridian).

Similarly, to deplete Soil, deplete the Lidui (ST45) point (the Metal point in the Stomach (Soil) meridian) and deplete the Shangqiu (SP5) point (Metal point in the Spleen (Soil) meridian). The book does not mention depleting the Metal point in Metal meridian (Lung meridian and Large intestine meridian).

Another difference from the original Five-element treatment principle is, to nourish one point, nourish its month point and the point that is supposed to restrain it at the same time. For example, stimulate the Yinbai (SP1) point (the Wood point in the Spleen (Soil) meridian).

This may not be a good choice of point, because Wood restrains Soil. It does not nourish the Soil meridian but restrains its energy flow. The author explains here that to use the Wood point on the Soil meridian is to transfer energy from the Wood point to the Soil point.

An additional difference is to use the great-grandmother point to nourish the great-grandson point (p101). For example, to stimulate a Soil point to nourish a Wood point, stimulate the Zhongfeng (LV4) point (Metal point) in the Liver (Wood) meridian first, then stimulate the Taiyuan (LU9) point (Soil point) in the Lung meridian (Metal meridian).

Let's have a look what would happen in such complex stimulation. First, to stimulate the Metal point in the Wood meridian, the Metal restrains the Wood. It does not nourish the Wood. Second, to stimulate the Soil point on the Metal meridian, the Soil point makes the Metal meridian stronger and the enhanced Metal meridian would restrain the Wood meridian even more, rather than nourish it!

This is the Nora "Five-element" acupuncture system. The author did not explain why it does not follow, or why omits, the principles of the original Chinese Five-element theory in the treatment plan.

The relationship between and among the five elements is the most important meaning of the Five-element theory. To separate things into five elements (groups) is to apply their relationships to solve problems. It is not for fun.

What would happen if we nourished one point (one meridian) but also restrained the same point (meridian)? To restrain one point (one meridian) again and again (according to the original Five-element theory), would result in a nourishing effect (according to the author)? Who is right and who is wrong? Both are right or both are wrong? At least we can make a summary that in this Five-element acupuncture, there is only nourishing and no depleting and no restraining. It almost means there is only Yang but no Yin. The Yin-Yang philosophic concept does not exist here.

In Chinese medicine, we can use nourishing and depleting at the same time. For example, we may nourish the Triple meridian (Fire meridian) but deplete the Heart shell meridian (also Fire meridian). They both belong to Fire meridians but they are different meridians and the energy movement direction in the two meridians is different (opposite). This is the way to spin the small circle (the Triple Jiao meridian and the Heart Shell meridian) smoothly.

2.3   Frequency and times of treatment

Any treatment needs proper treatment frequency and a total number of treatment sessions. However, frequency and the sessions required are usually not indicated in most of the textbook. This is understandable because different diseases, different people, and different acupuncture techniques need different treatment frequencies and total number of sessions. But in most of cases and for most of acupuncture styles, we need acupuncture once every day.

According to the Ren-yin and Mai-kou acupuncture system[4] introduced in the classic acupuncture book (named *Lingshu* and *Nanjing*), some kinds of pulse diagnosis require once a day of acupuncture; some need once every two days, and others need twice a day of acupuncture. There are no instructions for once every three days or more of acupuncture.
We have summarized the treatment frequency in acupuncture research done in Western countries. [4] It was found that in most of the research, the acupuncture was performed once or twice a week. We believe that the low treatment frequency in the Western countries is one of the possible reasons for the failure of the researchers to show positive results for acupuncture. We feel that it is very strange that acupuncture researchers in Western

---

[4] *Ren-yin and Mai-kou*: to feel pulse on the neck and on wrist respectively, so as to set up diagnosis of energy flow intensity in meridians. *Ren-yin*: pulse feels on neck. *Mai-kou*: pulse feels on wrist.

countries did not try to do acupuncture in closer frequency. Why do they believe that the healing effect of acupuncture can last for one week?

Here the author introduces that their acupuncture for most cases is once a week. (p93) Only for severe cases do they shorten the treatment interval. We feel that even for ordinary cases, once a week is too long in between sessions. Their healing result is in doubt.

2.4   Healing effect

The author said in the beginning of the book: "This style of Five-element acupuncture that I have been practicing and teaching is very simple but very practicable. To say it is simple: I believe that the most important rule in the nature is simple rather than more complex. After I deeply realized the Five-element, I found that it reveals the nature of life by so simple way. I experienced after my more than 20 years of studying and practice of the Five-element acupuncture that it can show the deep nature of life with a simple single line. It is so perfect. It transfers the understanding of life into detailed diagnosis and treatment procedures. The presence of the 'Dao" is proven by every session of the treatment." (p1)

"To deplete the 'Attached Spirit' is the most useful and most effective therapy of the Five-element acupuncture." (p135)

"Basically, it is very simple to correct the unbalanced left-right pulse, but it is very effective to save life." (p149) "Based on what I learned the use of Taixi (KD3) point, I use it as one of the acupuncture points to correct the unbalanced left-right pulse. It is indeed very useful." (p119)

The treatment of blockage between meridians is "very simple and very effective". (p153)

The treatment of blockage by scar tissue is "very simple". (p155)

"The aim of the transfer of energy Qi among meridians is to balance the Qi distribution among the element and organs. Such way of re-distribution helps to adjust the discrepancy among the 12 organs. It is simple to perform but the effect is very excellent. The Qi transfer therapy is one of the most powerful therapies, because it can balance the difference of the Qi and Blood among the five elements, so as to benefit all elements." (p97)

It seems that the author really found a very simple but very effective way of treatment for almost every disorder listed in the book. Is this really so?

The author wrote, "The healing effect is a long term, while the improvement of the disorders needs some length of time to show up. Every time of the treatment is to adjust the Qi and Blood little bit and little bit. Therefore there would have no major or abrupt changes in the Qi and Blood in the body. Therefore as a patient, we need patience." (p81)

"We can never predict what may happen after each treatment. Every patient has his or her own ways of reaction to the treatment. This is why it is complex. … We should give patient hope, but not guarantee." (p84)

"The reaction to the treatment is very different among patients, therefor we cannot predict what may happen and cannot plan the next step of the treatment." (p84)

"The diagnosis of the five element body constitution is extremely complex, it needs us, for a long time, to filter the signals from our sense organs and from other sources." (p88) "We must learn to sense very mild changes in the emotion of patients…." (p85)

"Acupuncturist every time needs to very careful to observe the tiny and slight changes in the body of the patients, and to make summary if the diagnosis of the dominated element of the patient is correct or not."

It seems that there is a lot of uncertainty about the results of treatments, because the change in body condition might not be so clear and that the acupuncturist needs to pay close attention to find very mild changes in patients.

Perhaps the author did not plan to have a major change after each treatment sessions, because she said, "The treatment needs several phases. Each phase is to reach a special aim. The first phase means the first several sessions of the treatments, including to select some acupuncture points to check the status of the Qi and Blood, then slowly nourish them. At this phase, choose the acupuncture points, the nature of which is the same as the dominated element of the body, but the stimulation should be very slight. This is because at the beginning of the treatment, the Qi and Blood of the patient is very unstable and very sensitive, the body can only be able to accept very mild stimulation." (p74) "If we look at an acupuncture point this way: it is from different angle/aspect to support the organ it is related. Every acupuncture point gives body a small order, asks the body to adjust itself. So, if we give too much order, it may disturb the body Qi and Blood… We may over-beat the acupuncture points to make them tired." (p81)

Is the Qi and blood of the patients really so fragile as to not be able to tolerate the amount of stimulation that can bring out clear improvement after each treatment? A slight stimulation will necessarily mean slight improvement?

According to the author, the healing effect of each session is difficult to predict or to expect, because the condition for each patient is different. The acupuncturist needs to be very careful to observe tiny changes in the patient, and check if the previous diagnosis of the dominant Element is correct or not.

Inner disorders could cause problems with the emotions of a patient (such as over happy, easy to get upset, continuous sad, frustrated feeling, frequent worry, easy to cry, etc.), as well as disorders in the autonomic nervous system (such as dizziness, headaches, insomnia, hot flashes, numbness in hands or feet, poor memory, irritated personality, disorder in menstruation, etc.).

In special cases, we might see hysteria. For these kinds of diseases, the treatment of the pre-treatment conditions can contribute to the improvement of the emotional disorders of the patient. Additionally some other procedures can also contribute to the improvement, such as the Jing point temperature test (it stimulates the Jing point on hands and feet), moxibustion before the Five-element needles and Primary point stimulation after Five-element needle stimulation.

Therefore the improvement in the emotion cannot be solely credited to the Five-element acupuncture per se.

More importantly, the deep compassion, deep talk with the patients, the expression of deep care about the patient, can all have placebo effect. The placebo effect as such might contribute much of the overall healing effect, because, as the author said, "only the warm created from mutual communication between the acupuncturist and the patient could improve the progress of the treatment. Without this, nothing can be obtained with the diagnosis and treatment." (p47)

The improvement of physical disorders prior to Five-element acupuncture can further enhance the placebo effect. It can also lead the acupuncturist to misunderstand that the dominant Element diagnosis of patient is correct.

As said by the author, the treatment actually starts once the acupuncturist meet the patient. Yes, this is true for the placebo effect. This type of acupuncture especially targets emotional disorders and patients with emotional disorders are more ready to be affected by another's care and compassion.

We normally think that improvement from a placebo effect would not happen quickly, nor reach a higher level of improvement and not last a long time. This is not true.

One of the placebo-containing surgical experiments showed that, a sham surgical operation on a group of patients with knee osteoporosis could reduce the pain to the same level as another group of similar patients with a typical operation. [5] In this experiment, the pain level reduced to 48.9±21.9 和 51.7±22.4, in both the sham group and the true operation group, respectively. Furthermore, the reduced pain could last the same length for both groups: two years.

Another study showed that a sham surgical operation can reduce migraine pain level by 57.7%.[6]

We have calculated that sham surgical operation can reduce pain level by 37% ± 18% (16 articles); [7] and sham Western medicine can have healing effect by 31%±18% (22 articles).

The intensity of the placebo effect in the sham group is very largely variable amongst patients. For some, their symptoms can be reduced by 100%. Those patients with strong emotional disorders are more affected by emotional intervention. Under the treatment of this Five-element emotional intervention, the improvement of emotional disorders in the patients would be fast and apparent. This is why the author emphasized the importance of the relationship with patients. But the improvement does not necessarily support the initial body Element diagnosis as correct.

According to the author, this Five-element acupuncture works more specifically for emotional disorders or its induced physical diseases. (p56). Is this its benefit over other styles of acupuncture? Yes and no.

This style of acupuncture can improve emotional disorders mostly, at least from its placebo effect, while other styles of acupuncture can also solve emotional disorders during the improvement of accompanied physical diseases. After treatment with most kinds of acupuncture, along with the improvement of physical disorders, patients usually also become calm and peaceful in mind and in mode. It is very common in acupuncture treatment that patients feel calm in the first session. The benefit for ordinary styles of acupuncture is that they do not require specific abilities of the acupuncturist such as sharp observation ability, good hearing and smelling ability, a very strong compassionate heart, or willingness to come into others' emotional lives. For acupuncturists who practice ordinary acupuncture, their healing effect is predictable and expectable for most cases.

The author admitted that, "It can be accepted that the healing by the Five-element acupuncture is from the inner side of the body towards the outside, while ordinary acupuncture improves body conditions from outside towards inside. All the styles of acupuncture work and their healing effects meet in the middle – because the outside and inner side should reach harmony." (p57) This means that this Nora Five-element acupuncture is not replacing ordinary styles of acupuncture. Other styles of acupuncture can also improve emotional disorders, while Nora Five-element acupuncture may not work as well in the improvement of physical diseases.

The treatment of typical mental diseases is a big challenge for ordinary styles of acupuncture, but also to Nora Five-element acupuncture because it would be hard to establish good relationship between the acupuncturist and the patient. In this case, the placebo effect would be hard to contribute to the healing effect. Disease information obtained from patient family members may not be trustworthy, so the diagnosis of the patient's body Element would be easy to get wrong.

What goal of acupuncture treatment can we reach, in order to change a patient's emotions, personality, and life attitude?

Some practitioners [8] say that acupuncture can change people's lives. For example, someone said that "The Five-element acupuncture is a very old and marvelous acupuncture therapy. It can not only improve physical diseases, but also the most mysterious thing is that it can adjust one's spirit. The so called spirit means one's emotion, personality, outlook on life (philosophy), sense of worth, etc.."

Is this style of acupuncture so powerful? It is possible to change emotions, to make someone calm down. But is it able to change their outlook on life and sense of worth? This might be beyond what it can really do. To change personality means to change a Fire person into Soil, into Metal, into Water or into Wood. Is this possible?

To have an emotional disorder means that the person is in an environment that does not match his dominant Element. For example a Wood person is in an environment which suppresses his personality, where everything needs to be done exactly according to rules, where most people dislike others who talk too much, or where the boss is a Metal person. Such an environment is not the one a Wood person likes, so he suffers from depression and unhappiness. Acupuncture treatment can only make him calm down, become more tolerable to the environmental stimuli and not so sensitive to environmental changes. We cannot change his environment and we cannot make him into a Metal person so that he feels comfortable in a Metal environment.

To completely or nearly completely make the person unaffected by the environment, we might need to change his view of life, and view of self worth. This may be only be achieved by religion.

In the book, we did not see chapters describing how to change a person's belief system so as to reach a change of their view of life and view of self worth, nor a chapter on how to discuss with the patient about his Element and its meaning to the patient. Most likely, we guess that the author must do so by herself with her patients. Such theory might be interesting, but may not be possible. To be able to change a patient's view of life might be overpraising the treatment method.

The author wrote, "The improvement usually needs some time to show up. Every time the Qi and Blood of the patient can be adjusted little bit, therefore we do not expect major difference due to abrupt disturbance of the Qi and blood. As patient, it is needed the patience…" (p81)

"… (with the healing results) we could never predict what may happen. The reaction to the treatment is variable among patients, so it is complex". "Every patient has different reaction, so we cannot predict their reaction so as to set up the treatment plan for the next time." (p84) "It is extremely complex for the Five-element diagnosis, it needs us for a quite long time to filter the sensitive signal from our sense organs." (p88)

This is how the author describes the healing effect of this style of acupuncture.

3   Discussion about some professional concept

3.1 On sense, not on logical analysis

The author emphasizes to "give up logical analysis of the information obtained, only depend on the sense." (p50) "This is because with logical thinking, it is easy to imagine the sense of the pulse into different feelings of the pulse. If your thinking changes, the pulse diagnosis will be changed accordingly. Doubt and influence by others could influence the evaluation of the pulse diagnosis." (p61)

This is different from any style of medicine. All medical systems, Chinese or Western, try to make the parameters for the diagnosis more objective, so that we can make the diagnosis the same from doctor to doctor. We try to reduce mistakes in the diagnosis affected by subjective guesses or senses. If every doctor/acupuncturist only depended on their own body senses to set up diagnosis, we could not have any case discussion, because the diagnosis by a given doctor would be entirely individual. How scary!

If we do not depend on pre-set parameters for diagnosis, how could we make the sensory diagnosis? For example, we may be able to make a guess for a person in front of us for his personality, willingness, good or evil spirit, even if the person we don't know or he has not spoken one word yet. But this is because we have set up the link for characteristics in the face and the personality, and we have practiced such predictions for a while and have had some experience. This is a natural course from unfamiliar to familiar and the practice makes us need less and less time to complete such prediction. We cannot force us not to use pre-set prediction knowledge in our mind.

In pulse diagnosis, we may feel that it is difficult to make the diagnosis, because the pulse might belong to this or that category of diseases. This is normal and this is a necessary step from unknown pulse diagnosis to expertise in diagnosis. The learning of any technique is as such. If we refuse such learning methods, no one would be able to achieve an expert level. (The author only senses a pulse as left-right imbalance and cannot link the pulse palpitation and the Five-element diagnosis. Does this suggest that the author did not have good logical practice in pulse diagnosis?)

The author said, "The signal emitted from the inner organs to the body surface can attract our attention quickly. If well trained, such quick reaction can be very powerful tool for the diagnosis. One of the advantages is it is not affected by complex thinking." (p49)

Note that the quick reaction requires the condition of "well trained" first.

"In the beginning, we found lots of various manifestations of the five elements in the body of patients. After we get more and more familiar to the characteristics of them, we can more clearly feel them and learn to store the various information collected from multiple sources, to be used for the next time of diagnosis. After we set up the information data bank about the five elements, we can more and more quickly find the manifestations of the five elements in ourselves and in the bodies we meet." (p50)

This suggests that the author admits that it is natural to get quicker diagnosis reactions by practicing again and again.

"Depending on sense only" might just reflect the difficulty in the diagnosis by the Five-element acupuncture system: the signal emitted from the inner organs to the body surface might not be strong enough; the sensitivity of the acupuncturist to such signal might not be sensitive enough; and the signal might not match the characteristics of known Five-elements. Any incompleteness in any of the steps could result in unreliable diagnosis.

"To increase sensation ability, to directly connect with self and others in emotion…requires us re-connect with the purest and the deepest side of our emotion. For those who have sufficient brave, it is the start to come into our own inner world and it is a real marvelous traveling experience." (50) "Therefore we need to spend time to re-learn the intuition of infants; evaluate emotion intuitionally; react to it intuitionally; and learn to avoid negative influence from ourselves to our patients." (p52) "In fact, all therapists should train themselves to have sharp ear as musicians; sharp vision as painter; sharp tongue and nose as cook; and to increase more and more our sensitivity to emotional signal." (p53)

How high the requirement for an acupuncturist (and for other kinds of therapist)! The requirement is superman. We do not know if the author and her teacher Warsley really have such super abilities.

3.2   Try not to stimulate the acupuncture points in the Heart meridian

The author warned not to use the acupuncture points in the Heart meridian (p101, 128, and 144). This is a very strange concept. In Chinese medicine, the Heart dominates the clearance of mind. This means it is responsible for the clear mode of the mind. For example, patients in coma and shock are not clear in the mind. We can tell that the Heart organ is disturbed in these patients. Also, many patients with mental diseases lost their "Heart" in the onset of the disease. But the emotion is associated with different organs too. For example, the Heart holds spirit; Lung holds bravery; Liver holds Hun; Spleen holds idea; and Kidney holds ambition. All of these belong to the broad concept of "Spirit". For example, if the Kidney is damaged, the patient may feel fear and have no desire to live. In this case, can we not stimulate the acupuncture points in the Kidney meridians?

To treat patients with emotional disorders, Traditional Chinese Medicine has never said that the acupuncture points in the Heart meridian should be avoided. We never learned from the historical record that acupuncture on the Heart meridian would make the emotional disease worse.

3.3   If the blood pressure difference is more than 40 mmHg, do not use moxibustion (p64, p115)

Our blood pressure has systolic pressure and diastolic pressure. The difference between the two pressures is called pressure difference.

To treat high blood pressure, we pay more attention to the nature of the patient body: if the body condition belongs to Hot, or Cold, to Phlegm, or Water, to Overwhelming or Deficiency. We do not pay much attention to the pressure difference. Based on the nature of the patient's body condition, we use or do not use moxibustion. If the patient's body belongs to Yang floating condition (severe condition of the Kidney deficiency), we still use moxibustion to "bring Yang back to its origin" and this is very efficient therapy. How should we worry that the moxibustion would increase blood pressure?

The normal range of the pressure difference is 30-40 mmHg. Once it is more than 60 mmHg, it is called enlarged pressure difference and, if it is less than 20 mmHg, narrowed pressure difference. [9] High blood pressure is diagnosed when the blood pressure is more than 140/90 mmHg. [10] According to this parameter, almost all hypertension patients have enlarged pressure difference. Should we say that almost all patients with high blood pressure should not be given moxibustion treatment?

Rong W (2013) [11] tested the effects of moxibustion treatment on high blood pressure. They randomly separated 160 cases of primary hypertension patients into two groups, 80 cases in each. For the treatment group, they used ordinary medicine plus moxibustion for one month, and in the control group, the ordinary medicine only. They found that in the experiment group with moxibustion, both systolic and diastolic pressure were reduced dramatically, as compared with the control group (p<0.05). They commented that moxibustion works to reduce hypertension. In this study, 20 cases belong to Liver Yang overwhelming, 24 cases belong to Qi-blood deficiency, and 36 cases belong to Kidney essence. Before treatment, the systolic pressure was 100-150 mmHg, the average 139.03±12.39 mmHg, and diastolic pressure was 60-100 mmHg, the average 80.85±9.16 mmHg. Apparently the pressure difference was more than 40 mmHg and moxibustion works for all types of hypertension.

Daoxia S (2016)[12] and Yaqiu L (2014) [13] also reported on the use of moxibustion in the treatment of elderly hypertension. After treatment the stability of blood pressure in the treatment groups was higher than the control groups, but the incidence of complication due to hypertension was dramatically lower in the treatment groups than in the control groups. They did not indicate side effects due to the use of moxibustion.

3.4   Body constitution

There are ways in China to tell the Five-element body constitution but they are mostly not based on person's way of talking, willingness, voice, skin color or body odor. They are mostly based on body shape and characteristics on the face [14,15] and hands.[16,17] That means they use more objective parameters to tell the difference between someone's Five-element category. We call it face prediction and hand prediction technique.

For example, for a Wood type of person, [18] their body is slim and straight, with projected bones; the face is broad upper and narrow in the chin; skin color is blue-pale tint; the voice has a high pitch; the personality is compassionate, warm, and forgiving, but the will is easy to shift.

A Water person has the following characteristics: big and round body shape; bones are not projected; looks like they have a lot of muscle (fat); thick back; round back; big and coarse eyebrows; big eyes; face is slightly dark in color; voice changes slow or fast; the personality is rich in feelings, rich in senses; they are rich in imagination; clever; lovely; physical motion is not restricted by a big body. The shape of hands also matches the shape of the body.

For a Wood person, the hands are thin and long (good for playing piano). For Water, hands are thick in the palm.

Therefore, even if the person stands 2 meters away without speaking a word, the future teller can, after some practice, tell the personality of the person. The accuracy of such a prediction is not largely variable from teller to teller. Though it is listed here with the different skin color/tints, and voice, they are normally not the primary parameters to tell person's personality.

In the Nora Five-element acupuncture system, the acupuncturist and the patient must have verbal communication, we must ask the patient about his or her life history and life environment, we must observe the skin color and tint and smell body odor, all to make diagnosis. The parameters used here are easy to be cloudy and vague. It is difficult to result in a quick diagnosis.

In Western countries, it is much easier (than in China) to meet dark colored people. It is not easy to tell the difference in the skin color among different people. The body odor is also easily confused with the use of perfume, herbal lotion, and a person's own body odor. Therefore, the parameters needed for the body Element constitution diagnosis in Nora Five-element acupuncture are not reliable.

3.5   Body constitution as disease diagnosis

During the diagnosis in Chinese medicine, no matter if it is herbal therapy or acupuncture, the information obtained reflects the current body condition, not congenital information about the body. Though we also access body constitution, such as Shaoyin body, Jueyin body, Taiyin body, or Yin-deficiency body, Yang-deficiency body, Phlegm-wetness body; or Guizhi (name of a herb) Tang body, Huangqi (name of a herb) tang body, all also reflect the current body condition.

These body constitution diagnoses are also used as a reference, not a definite decisive guide for treatment. For example, when we face a Huangqi [5] body condition in a patient (such as obesity, pale skin color, easy to have swelling on leg and pain in the knee, etc.), we still need to make an exact diagnosis for the patient's current nature of the disease. If the current problem is a cough, then we still need make sure which kind of cough the patient has this time and we may not really add the herb Huangqi in the formula for the treatment of current cough. Only when there is no extra problem do we start to care about the treatment of the Huangqi constitution.

We do not know when the ancient Chinese made the Five-element body constitution the target of treatment with acupuncture or with herbal therapy. But, Five-element theory has never been lost from the Chinese acupuncture system. It is not for the treatment of body constitution, but for given diseases.

---

[5] Huangqi: name of a kind of herb.

Body constitution changes along with age. The body constitution of a person is not only one Element, but the mixture of two or more elements. Otherwise, can we say that there are only five kinds of people in the world and we can guess the personality of every famous politician in the world?

In Chinese face prediction, we are very careful to identify the mixture of the body constitution and the relationship of the Element in a person to predict the person's future. This is the marvelous nature of Chinese face prediction.

Let us see an example. The dominant Element of Chinese prime minister Li could be Metal but his skin is dark. Dark is Water, Water is the son of the Metal, so it can be said that the dark color for Mr. Li is not a bad sign. If someday his face or skin turns red, something bad might have happened to him. Red is Fire. Fire restrains Metal. If someday he suffers cough and he is very busy with work, according to Five-element theory, we should deplete the Heart meridian, not nourish the Metal. This is because the stress in the work (Fire) restrains his respiratory system (Metal). If his cough happens usually after eating too much, we should nourish the Spleen (Soil) system. If the cough is with lots of phlegm, we need to deplete the Kidney meridian (Water). If the cough happens in Spring, or the pulse on the Liver position is too strong, we may deplete the Liver meridian. Only when there is no clear sign for Heart Fire, Liver Wood, Spleen Soil or Kidney water, should we consider to nourish the Lung Metal.

This is the way we use Five-element theory for treatment, even though the body constitution stays the same. Therefore, to apply the Five-element theory in medical treatments, we should pay attention to the relationship between the five elements. If we practice Five-element theory as the author did, always nourishing one element and "conducting" energy from other meridians to one meridian, and not caring about the relationship of nourish, restrain, further-restrain and reverse restrain, this is not typical or original Five-element theory.

The importance and usefulness of the Five-element theory is that it reveals the relationship between the elements. To separate the things into five groups is not for fun at all. After erasing the complex relationship between the elements, the Five-element theory becomes meaningless.

In the same way, that we separate things into Yin and Yang is to reveal the relationship between the Yin and Yang, that the Yang can transform into Yin, that Yin can transform into Yang, and that Yang is the dominant force and the Yin is relatively a follower (This is not the same concept as Chairman Mao said). If we do not pay attention to the mutual transformation and the influence on each other, what is the use for the Yin and Yang concept? From this point of view, we believe that to omit the relationship between the Five elements is not at all a development of the original Five-element theory, but a distortion of it. We really wish that the author could tell us if anyone has done a comparison study on such modified Five-element theory without caring if the restrain and reverse-restrain relationship between elements would work better than the original Five-element theory.

This acupuncture system separates body constitution into five dominant element types, omits the co-existing other types of element, and focuses the treatment just on the dominant element. Even if the correction of the dominant element is a success, the co-existing elements were not taken into consideration for correction yet. The author presumes that once the dominant element is corrected, its energy will be generously distributed to other elements. How do we know this is true in nature? It almost means that the Summer will share its heat to the Fall and to the Winter, that the Spring will re-distribute its upper-rising energy to the Fall when it needs down-descending energy! The author's presumption confuses the different and unique nature of the Elements.

3.6   How to understand the Five-element theory

The author understands the meaning of the five elements as, "The five Shu points add into the organ it associated, the nature of five elements. For example, the Metal point on the Fire meridian (Heart, Small intestine, Heart Shell and Three Jiao) makes the Fire as Metal nature, the hard as metal; the Soil point on the Water meridian (Kidney, Urine bladder) can make the water as hard and nourish." (p125)

What does it mean to make the Fire hard and to make the Water hard? It is difficult to understand.

"We nourish the dominated element by transferring meridian Qi to it, by transferring extra Qi in other meridians to it. After the Qi in the dominated meridian is full and it returns into the dominated status in the body, it would generously share its own Qi to other meridians (organs); if the dominated element is in struggle for survival, it needs help from other elements. Once it gets recovered, other elements also get relaxed." (p98)

This is how the author understands the meaning of the five elements. They have a mutual help and nourish relationship, not a restrain relationship, because "The acupuncture points that we choose, if they match the same as the element of the body dominant, the sequence in use of them and the healing nature of them is not so important for the healing effect. The importance is to give continuous nourishment to the dominated element through all acupuncture points on the same element meridian (organ). This is as to add a brick to the hall each time the acupuncture point is used." (p77)

This means that once the acupuncture points are on the same element meridian as the dominant body element, the stimulation of them would work to have a healing effect. The difference among the five element points in the same meridian does not matter too much for the overall healing effect.

However, our understanding of the five elements in each meridian is that the five element acupuncture points on each meridian adjust the speed and stability of Qi flow in the meridian.

This means that with the mutual function of the five element points, the Qi flow in the meridian is stable, smooth and consistent. It makes the Qi flow not too fast this time but slow next time, not too big this time but too small next time. This is like a car: the car stands on the Primary point. In the Kidney meridian, it is the Water point. The Water point is its starting point (ignite). The Wood point is used to speed up the Qi flow (Water nourish the Wood). The Fire point slows down the car (it works as a resistant to the car, so the Water needs to restrain the Fire in normal situation). The Soil point is the brake (Soil restrains the Water normally) and the Metal point supplies fuel to the Water (Metal is the mother of the Water).

In this way, the car can run smoothly with abrupt jumps from time to time (balanced condition). This is the micro-adjustment mechanism in each meridian. Therefore, once an acupuncture point of the five element points is stimulated, it would either promote the Qi flow, or slow down the flow.

For example, if we nourish the Fire point on Metal meridian, it would slow down the Qi flow in the Metal meridian, because nourishment of the Fire makes the Fire point functions strongly restrain the Metal meridian (increase the brake function). If we deplete the Fire point to reduce its brake function, the Qi flow in the Metal meridian would be increased (the restraining force is reduced).

This concept is also applicable to the five element meridians. Through the mutual nourish and restraining relationship among the five element meridians, the Qi flow in the whole body is also smooth and stable.

Therefore, to erase the mutual helping and mutual restraining relationship between the five element acupuncture points (and meridians), and only to stimulate other element points or meridians with the hope of supplying the dominant meridians, is done to make things simple, it may not be the development of Five-element theory but may twist and misunderstand it.

3.7 Relationship between the meridians with the surface-inner relationship

The author regards the some element acupuncture points/meridians as the same. For example, Kidney and Urine bladder meridian both belong to Water meridian. To nourish the dominant Water body element, both the Kidney meridian and the Urine meridian (they have a surface-inner relationship) would be nourished at the same time. For Fire dominant body element, the four Fire meridians would be nourished: Heart meridian, the Small intestine meridian (the Heart and the Small intestine meridian have a surface-inner relationship), the Heart Shell meridian and the Three Jiao meridian (the Heart Shell and the Three Jiao meridian have a surface-inner meridian).

Actually, the relationship between the surface meridian and the inner meridian is not just to conduct each other to share the Qi flow between them. As having been clearly explained by "Si Shen Xin Yuan" theory, the Qi flow in the surface-inner couple meridians is opposite. For example, the Qi in the Stomach is to fall (descending) and that in the Spleen is to rise (Ascending). The Qi movement in the surface-inner couple meridian is also a circle. If the descending force is too strong, the ascending Qi would be too weak. For example, if the Stomach Qi is too strong (descending Qi), the Spleen Qi (Ascending Qi) will be low. Therefore, to nourish the surface-inner related couple meridian the same time obscures the meaning of the surface-inner relationship.

In the treatment of the dominant body element, the author always regards that the reason for the sickness is the weakness (deficiency) of the dominant body element, so she tries to find the dominant element meridian and to nourish it. According to what we mentioned above, if the dominant body element, which is always attached to solid organ meridians, such as the Heart, Liver, Lung, Spleen and Kidney, not hollow organs such as Small intestine, etc., is weak, then the Qi in the corresponding hollow organ meridian would be too strong. For example, in a dominant Water body, we should nourish the Kidney meridian to improve the Qi flow in it, and at the same time we need to deplete the Qi flow in the Urine bladder meridian. This is the traditional Chinese way to balance the Qi flow in the meridians with a surface-inner relationship. In this example, we must nourish two points in the Kidney meridian but deplete one point in the Urine bladder meridian, as indicated in our acupuncture bible book.

3.8   To insert needle on left first is to nourish; and to insert needle on right is to deplete

There are various techniques to reach a nourishing or a depletion result of acupuncture stimulation, such as with different way of twisting, pulling or inserting, following breath in or out, following or against the direction of energy flow in the meridians, etc. But we have no concept that, to insert a needle on the left would be nourishing and to insert a needle on the right would be depleting. In the book, it is said that to insert a needle on left first is to nourish and to insert needle on right is to deplete. (p110) We want to know where such nourish-depletion technique comes from and how it works.

In most Chinese styles of acupuncture, we may also be concerned about acupuncture on the left or the right. The left or right side is more related to gender, e.g. male or female.

For example in one of the Hand acupuncture systems, the corresponding body limbs in the four fingers are different in males and females.

In Ghost-13 needle acupuncture, we start needles first on the left side for male and first on the right side for female.

In Classical acupuncture system (The Pan's Classical system – Old Acupuncture Book-induced Acupuncture System), it is said that the direction of energy flow in meridians in males and females is different, so the sequence of acupuncture would also be different. For males, insert the needle on the left side first on the arm (on leg, do the right first), and for females, insert the needle the right side first on the arm (on leg, the left side first).

Therefore, the left-right concept is related to the male-female, even to the time of the day (before or after noon). Acupuncturist should know that the direction of the energy flow in the meridians is different in males and females (this is not indicated in many Acupuncture Textbooks). Therefore, if inserting needles on the left side for male is nourishing, then it should be depletion for female.

3.9 Non-retention of needle is nourishing and leaving the needle is depleting

It is important to consider whether to leave the needle or not in acupuncture treatment. The retention time is related to the healing effect for different diseases. Even different people with the same type of disease (TCM concept disease) need different times of retention. For some types of acupuncture, there is no retention time at all, no matter if it is overwhelming condition (supposed to have depletion) or deficiency condition (supposed to have nourishing technique). From the Classical acupuncture point of view, for Hotness condition (Fire condition) the needle is not retained but for Cold condition, the needle should be kept in the spot for some time.

For Nora Five-element acupuncture, whenever the nourishing technique is needed, moxibustion was performed on the acupuncture point first. The moxibustion has already stimulated the acupuncture point before the insertion of the needle. The total time of the stimulation of the acupuncture point is not short. How can we say that when the needle was not retained it is nourishing?

3.10   Following the Qi flow direction is nourishing and against its flow direction is depleting (p110)

We agree that this is a correct way in Chinese acupuncture treatment.

The point here is that we must know the direction of the Qi flow in the body.

According to the acupuncture text book, the Qi moves: for the three Hand Yang meridians, from chest to hand; three Hand Yin meridians from hand to head; for the three Foot Yang meridians, from head to foot; and for three Yin Foot meridians, from foot to chest.

According to the explanation in the Pan Xiaochuan Acupuncture system for the Acupuncture bible, this is the way of Qi flow for males for the left side of the body and before the noon. The flow direction on the right side of the body in males is opposite. This is also the way for females on the right side of the body and after noon.

Such flow sequence is not introduced in acupuncture textbooks, nor in the Nora Five-element acupuncture book. If the direction of the Qi flow is unclear, how can we perform the following-against following nourish and depletion techniques of acupuncture?

3.11   Treatment of "Attached Spirit"

"Attached spirit" means some extra energy body comes in and attaches to the body of the patient. There are different kinds of "Attached spirit", and not all of them are bad for the patient. One such spirit comes into the body of the patient for the aim to use the body to express its sadness and unhappiness, and it wants to speak out about what it wants. Acupuncturists need to know this (because this kind of information is not included in Acupuncture textbook), know how to communicate with the "spirit", understand the reasons of the attachment, and to know how to meet the need and the request of the "spirit". Unless the "spirit" sticks in the body and refuses to leave, the acupuncturist does not use strong stimulation by acupuncture to force it to leave. If the acupuncturist does not have such training, or has never seen how some others deal with it, it is better not dealing with such a case.

Information on attached spirit is as follows: [19]

> Today we are going to introduce the Ghost-13 needle therapy in Chinese acupuncture. It sound very much of superstition, but it works well. It can help the recover the patient who has had "extra spirit" attached in the body. This therapy is summarized earliest by Dr. Sun Simiao, using Chinese medicine way of diagnosis, perform acupuncture on "13 Ghost" acupuncture points, to treat insomnia, depression, anxiety, schizophrenics. The result is excellent. The recurrence rate is low.

> ……

> After remember the pithy formula, now we continue to introduce the location of the acupuncture points and the way of acupuncture. First of all, we need to make sure that the person is indeed attached by "extra spirit". We can use our thumb and point finger to pitch the sides of the root stem of middle finger of the patient. If we can

feel strong pumping, it means there is attachment of "extra spirit". If not, it means that the condition belongs to epilepsy.

The 13 Ghost points are: Renzhong (DU26), Shaoshang (LU11), Yinbai (SP1), Daling (PC7), Shenmai (UB62), Fengfu (DU16), Jiache (ST6) , Chengjiang (REN24), Laogong (PC8), Shangxing (Du23), Huiyin (REN1), Quchi (LI11), and middle under the tongue.

1) Advise first. For example, face the patient, you can say: who you are? Where are you from? Are you persecuted to death? Tell me what you want? I can try my best to meet your need. You want to eat or drink? You want meat, or money or something else? If you want money, I can burn money to you. All in all, I can meet your request…

2) After you tell it this way, the ghost may start to talk with you. If it brings out some request, you first answer yes to help. Ask the patient family to do what it wants and burn money to it. It means to respect it.

3) If you have tried to communicate with it again and again but it does not talk to you and ignores you, then you can start to force it. You can take out needle to scare it. If this does not work, then you really insert needle to punish it.

4) Acupuncture: commonly used needles are ordinary thin needle, triple-edge needle, and plum needle. After insert of the needle, first to slight stimulate, while threaten the "spirit" if it obeys and gives up. If it agrees to discuss conditions for it to leave, discuss with it and do it as it asks. If it refuses to give up, then start strong stimulation. The needle can be twist strongly with big circle, or insert-and-pulling quickly and deeply, or shaking the needle strongly.

Usually one acupuncture point as Shaoshang (LU11) is sufficient. You can also choose additional two or three other acupuncture points from the 13 Ghost point group.

Specific remind:

1) The article here is for brief introduction about the use of "13 Ghost" acupuncture technique. To use it, please consult with professional acupuncturist. Without really understand Chinese medicine and have no any practical experience, no understanding about the "13-Ghost" acupuncture system, better not to do it. Otherwise, you have to take responsibility by yourself.

2) During treatment, follow the ancient principle to always leave a way for the "spirit" to leave, e.g. do not force it to the corner. Remember: try not to use the acupuncture point under the tongue, the Huiyin (REN1) and the Renzhong (DU26) points. Other acupuncture points in the 13-Ghost group can also work and can leave it a way to leave. Even if it has been controlled by you and it leaves, you still need to respect it by finishing whatever you and the patient family promised it, such as burning paper money and so on.

3) During the treatment by professional acupuncturists, it is better to bring and hold a "Protecting signal" in the acupuncturist's body, so as to prevent the "spirit" may retaliate back. Whenever the acupuncturist is sick, weak, or the body Yang Qi is not sufficient, do to perform this type of treatment.

4) The "13-Ghost" acupuncture is not perfect for everything. It only works for some specific condition and the result is closely related to the body energy level of the acupuncturist as well. Patient is recommended to go to professional medical institute, not just try quack doctor.

There are also other ways for the diagnosis and treatment of "Attached spirit" [20,21,22,23]

According to the theory above, it is necessary to make sure if there really is an "Attached spirit" inside the body of patient. If the answer is yes, it is necessary to have good communication with the "Attached spirit" and regulate the resentment relationship between the "Attached spirit" and the concerned patient or patient family members. It is not good to involve oneself in such sensitive thing abruptly and carelessly. It is necessary to protect oneself during the treatment. All of these were not mentioned in the Nora book. It seems that it is the same to treatment for "Attached spirit" as in treating any other kinds of disease.

In the treatment of "Attached spirit", the author asked patients to tell if there is Deqi sensation in the acupuncture (p139). In reality, when the patient is affected by the "Attached spirit", it is the "Attached spirit" who talks with the acupuncturist. The patient has lost consciousness and cannot talk with the acupuncturist. Acupuncture is what the "Attached spirit" fears and dislikes. How can the acupuncturist ask the "Attached spirit" to co-operate with the acupuncturist to answer his question? Is the "Attached spirit" that we mean here not the same as the "Attached spirit" that the author means?

In the diagnosis of "Attached spirit", the pulse is not used, but in the treatment, it is necessary that acupuncturist should pay attention to the eye spirit and the pulse of the patient. What might the pulse be, before and after the treatment?

The treatment of the "Attached spirit" seems not difficult, because "During the first session of treatment, if you have been very careful and paid much attention to make sure that all the acupuncture points achieved Deqi sensation", "it is very rare that the "Attached Spirit" cannot be depleted". (p140) If this is true, the treatment of mental diseases, including hysteria, should not be difficult to cure?

3.12   Treatment of "Imbalanced left-right pulse"

The author says, "Basically, it is very simple and easy to correct the imbalance of left-right pulse, but it can really save life. If such imbalance is not corrected, the King organ (the heart) would crash down due to heavy burden and cause stop of life. Once the diagnosis is set up… it should be treated as soon as possible. Otherwise the patient might die." (p149) According to the treatment plan recommended, it indeed seems that the treatment is not complex. It is possible to correct such pulse by performing acupuncture on 7-8 acupuncture points in one session, because it is said, "if the pulse was not correct by one session, repeat it next time. See, it can be expected to correct such risk pulse condition in just one session." (p149)

The imbalanced left-right pulse may not be so dangerous to life. In the book *Yi Xue Zhong Zhong Can Xi Lu*, there is an herbal formula for the treatment of Liver deficiency with pain in the legs. Patients with such diseases have a typical pulse pattern where the left pulse is less than the right pulse. In a clinic, such left-right imbalanced pulse is not at all rare and it may not be so easy to correct, because it involves three organs: Heart, Liver, and Kidney.

Imbalanced left-right pulse should belong to Mai-kou pulse type. It means that the left three pulses are weaker than the right three pulse in males. According to Pan's Classical acupuncture system[6], if the left is weaker than the right, it belongs to Mai-kou pulse; but in females, it is Ren-ying pulse. The principle in the acupuncture treatment is quite different.

The really dangerous pulse condition should be when the pulse in both sides are very thin and weak (the Shaoyin pulse). The author did not mention this type of the pulse.

3.13   Acupuncture based on pulse diagnosis

Not many acupuncture systems are based on pulse diagnosis. One of them is Pan's Classical acupuncture system. It emphasizes the importance of pulse diagnosis in the practice of acupuncture, and does not mention the specific requirement of excellent acupuncturist-patient relationship. In fact, with this type of Five-element acupuncture, even if there is no verbal communication between the acupuncturist and the patient, the acupuncture can be started after pulse diagnosis. This is because this system believes that any illness in the body could be reflected in the pulse. Correction of the pulse would be able to solve the illness. Knowing what's wrong from the pulse, acupuncture can be started. According to the followers of this acupuncture system, it seems true.

In Pan's acupuncture system, the meaning of the pulse is different for male and for female. During pulse palpitation, the acupuncturist should be very quiet and keep a neutral mind, rather than asking the pulse 'Small intestine, what you need today?', or 'Heart, what you need today?'. (p60) For the pulse palpitation, we find the shallow-floating pulse, so the finger touches the skin very lightly. If there is no such shallow-floating pulse, then we try

---

[6] Note of lecture.

to find deep-weak pulse. It is much easier to master the technique than with textbook pulse diagnosis.

According to the introduction by Dr. Pan, there are three kinds of pulse diagnosis system in China: the Qi-hua pulse; Micro-pulse and Taisu pulse. The Qi-hua pulse is used to test the status of the Qi and Blood circle in the body; the Micro-pulse can find specific diseases such as gall stone; Taisu pulse can test the current and future of life, such as personality, marriage situation, etc. For the latter two, it is hard to master but it shows that it is possible to know people's personality by pulse.

In treatment, Pan's Classical acupuncture system pays much attention to the dynamic direction of the Qi flow. It can be different for male and for female, left side or right side of the body, and the time (before noon or after noon). For the nourishing technique, insert the needle at a small angle to the skin and insert it shallowly (very shallow too). For the depletion technique, insert the needle at a larger angle (about 30 degrees) and insert it deeply. We also apply the nourish-depletion technique according to the breath of patients. We pay attention to the balance between the surface-inner couple meridian that the Qi in one meridian is ascending and another one is descending. The dominant disease list is very broad, not restricted if the disease is caused by inner or outer factors, and not restricted if it is a physical problem or an emotional disorder. All of these are different from Nora Five-element acupuncture.

3.14   Relationship between the personal Element of the author and the Five-element acupuncture system here

So far, we have found some relationship between the author's body dominant element and her Five-element acupuncture. The dominant element of the author could be Fire. This has been admitted by the author herself, because the Fire is her "Domain". The Fire is her "House yard", among the five elements. Fire is open, warm, seeking "Big vigor and vitality", and big influence. The weakness however is that the person is unstable, has no shape to follow, and is not careful. This is largely different from Metal, where Fire dislikes the Metal for its following rules and doing things carefully.

During reading the chapter for diagnosis, we found that the description for the characteristics of each element is very literary, but there are no distinguishing marks to identify each element. The book never talks about what we should do if we notice characteristics indicating more than two elements. In the treatment, the treatment principle is shortened to just using the nourishing-mother and depleting-son in the same meridian, not between meridians.

It does not care about nourish, restrain, reverse restrain, or such commonly used relationships among the five elements. The complex relationship among the five elements is simplified into just help each other: if one meridian is sick, we can conduct energy from other meridians to nourish it. After it has been nourished to normal, it would also ready to share its energy to others.

Treatment uses pulse palpitation, and can identify the left-right different pulse, but not more types of pulses, such as when the left pulse stronger than right pulse, if both Cun positions are stronger than both Chi positions, and it does not say that we should take time to identify if any individual position is stronger or weaker.

Treatment uses the Jing point temperature test, but it stimulates all the Jing points, and cannot stimulate only a small number of the acupuncture points.

Treatment uses the stimulation on left first as nourishing technique and on right as depletion technique, not the most commonly used acupuncture nourish-depletion technique (because these techniques take time?). Doing moxibustion before acupuncture and using Primary points at the end of every session makes it seem that the author does not feel confident about the Five-element acupuncture.

The author says that, after several treatments, if the acupuncture points match the body element, the sequence of the acupuncture points and the nature of the acupuncture points are not so important for the final results.

The important thing is using various acupuncture points on the dominant meridian to continuously nourish it. So, the nature of each acupuncture point is not important? The separation of acupuncture points as five elements is not important?

All of these suggest that the treatment is a broad-targeting therapy. It is like using a shotgun to shoot a bird: even if the bird cannot be shot down, we can hurt it. Treatment uses various methods, and does not care about details in the requirement for each. What the author pays much attention to is the good relationship with patients, not the acupuncture per se. Talking with patients is what the Fire person likes because it is fun. The good relationship (a kind of placebo effect) can bring about some healing effects, and the following acupuncture procedures seemingly do not bring noticeable contribution to the healing effect.

4 Discussion

Based on analysis above, we find that the Nora Five-element system is new (compared with Traditional Chinese medicine), that it targets the correction of so-called dominant body element of the patient, and that it takes the improvement of emotion of patient as its main goal of treatment.

For this acupuncture system, the majority of the healing effect comes from a good relationship between the acupuncturist and patient. As the author says, without such good relationship, none of the later treatments would work. Such a good relationship should work for all kinds of the disorders of the body elements, so it is non-specific effect.

The healing effect, if any, could be attributed to treatments that do not belong to the Five-element acupuncture per se, such as (1) the Jing point temperature test (it stimulates all the Jing points on feet or hands during the test); (2) treatment for "Attached spirit", "AE", imbalanced left-right pulse, blockage of energy flow between the meridians, blockage between scar tissues; (3) moxibustion before each Five-element acupuncture; (4) stimulation of the Primary acupuncture points after each session.

Nora Five-element acupuncture technique does not follow the application principles of the original Five-element theory[7]. Therefore it is a modified

"Five-element theory". We are interested to know if anyone has ever compared the two kinds of Five-element theory, to see if the relationship between the elements in the original Five-element theory is useless, or if the modified Five-element is a simpler or more powerful treatment. Because the healing effect of the Nora Five-element acupuncture has been largely taken over by other ways of acupuncture listed above, whether it works or not becomes less important. In addition, any of the acupuncture treatments, if they do improve physical problems, can enhance the placebo effect already attributed to the "good relationship" between the acupuncturist and patient.

All in all, it appears that, even if the Five-element body constitution is clearly established (it is difficult actually, as the author says), subsequent treatments (including a good relationship) are non-specific. It is hard to tell that it is the Five-element acupuncture that stimulates a specific element of meridian and that it works for the corresponding element body constitution, because there are so many non-specific treatments before and after it.

Our suspicions may or may not be correct. We strongly recommend a comparison study to compare Nora Five-element acupuncture with any of the most popular styles of current acupuncture. We need to know to what extent this Five-element acupuncture works because of the "good relationship between the acupuncturist and patient", and if the modified Five-element acupuncture really works better than the original Five-element acupuncture.

Such a comparison study might be difficult. It is not hard to find an expert level acupuncturist who practices ordinary acupuncture, but it is indeed

---

[7] The principle in the choice of acupuncture points in the Five-element acupuncture might be influenced very much by Japanese style acupuncture (said by the author). We do not know the Japanese acupuncture at all. It might be very different from the original Five-element theory used in China by Chinese. However, according to our understanding of the bible book for acupuncture, the book Lingshu and Nanjing, the original acupuncture does not stimulate the mother point and the son point on the same meridian, nor to stimulate the mother meridian and the son meridian at the same time. To nourish and to deplete the same point (or the same meridian) is not the common way of the Five-element theory (though in some other acupuncture system may do so unconsciously.)

hard to find an expert level acupuncturist who practices Nora modified Five-element acupuncture. Beside the requirement that the patients are willing to have deeper communication with acupuncturists (better to be body element of Wood, Fire or Soil), the acupuncturists have to also be willing to come deep into the patient's emotional life. In addition, the acupuncturist must have super abilities such as sharp vision, hearing, smelling, intuition, etc.

Even if we are lucky enough to find such as expert, we have to also completely follow the treatment schedule recommended by the author, without any change or modification, including having acupuncture once a week for 6 to 8 sessions. Also, to test the efficiency of the modified Five-element acupuncture, the healing effect from other treatments (such as the treatment for "Attached spirit", "AE", imbalanced pulse, etc.) should be isolated and excluded.

If we are not able to find such as expert Nora Five-element acupuncturist, this type of acupuncture will be like the "Emperor's new clothing" forever.

Luckily, we found one such study. It was published by Paterson C (2011).[24] The author allocated 80 patients into two groups: a Five-element acupuncture group and a control group. Both groups were given basic Western medicine treatments in the same way. The patients suffered from medically unexplained symptoms. 51% of them suffered from musculoskeletal disorders, 13% had emotional issues, 10% had headaches, and 10% had chronic fatigue.

The Five-element acupuncture was performed by 8 Five-element acupuncturists. It was performed once a week (one hour each session) initially, then once every two weeks, and later once every month, for a total of 12 sessions and for 26 weeks. The treatment was individualized. The main index for the treatment result is the MYMOP and others (see Table 1). After 23 treatments, the MYMOP index reduced in the Nora acupuncture group from 4.3 to 3.3 (reduced by 23%) and in the control group from 4.6 to 4.0 (down by 13%), with no significant difference statistically. The maximum index in the MYMOP is 6. If we transfer it into normal 10 scales, it means that in the acupuncture group, the symptom level was reduced from 7.1 down to 5.5 and, in the control group, from 7.6 down to 6.6. Even if it reached significance statistically, it means that the acupuncture treatment reduced symptoms from 6.6 to 5.5 only.

If Chinese acupuncturists in China treated similar patients 12 times and they only reduced the symptoms by 23%, they would feel shame for allowing patients to spend their time and money on such results. However, for such results, the author summarized, "The addition of 12 sessions of five-element acupuncture to usual care resulted in improved health status and wellbeing that was sustained for 12 months."

Once the article was published, it triggered very hot debate that this is a very strongly misleading article. One of the most famous opponents is David Colquhoun.[25] David published an article before that said acupuncture is merely a placebo. [26] For his article, we have written an article too and pointed out the errors and mistakes in the acupuncture research in Western countries. 4 However, here we agree with David that in this Five-element acupuncture study, the Five-element acupuncture did not exercise its supposed healing effect at all; no clear placebo effect can be seen!

We feel that the reasons for the failure of this study could be:

(1) The Five-element technique is not a working style of acupuncture. Not to say that it does not work for disorders of physical sources.

(2) The interval between the treatment sessions is too long. This is typical for most acupuncture research in Western countries and this is one of the major reasons for the failure of most acupuncture studies.
(3) The clinical skill of the acupuncturists in the study was not ensured.

Acupuncture therapy moved from China to other countries, from one country to another. Many things have been modified, resulting in Korea acupuncture, Japanese acupuncture, Western acupuncture, etc. We call the Five-element acupuncture examined here UK Five-element acupuncture or Nora Five-element acupuncture. This is so that we can tell the difference between the various styles of acupuncture.
It is clear that the Nora Five-element acupuncture has quite a few modifications from the original Five-element theory in acupuncture. For

all such modifications, if the author cannot give reasons for the modification, it may not be a "development" of acupuncture, but rather it could be a damage or distortion of acupuncture. It seems to make the Five-element theory easier to use, but it may also reduce the actual healing effect of the original Five-element acupuncture. The fact that it emphasizes very much the effect of the good relationship between the acupuncturist and the patient in the cure of diseases makes us strongly suspect that this type of acupuncture, even the whole acupuncture system, gives a placebo effect only.

Finally, we have to admire the beautiful writing of the author, who put a beautiful picture in front of us, showing the colorful five element body constitutions. It made me forget that it is a professional guide book while reading, feeling more like an interesting and attractive novel. After putting down the book, what I remembered most is the five element figures, but I cannot separate them from each other.

I also admire the nice translation by Chinese acupuncturist, Long Mei, for her deep and nice Chinese language level and high skill in translation. From her translation, I can imagine how beautiful the original English version of the book might be.

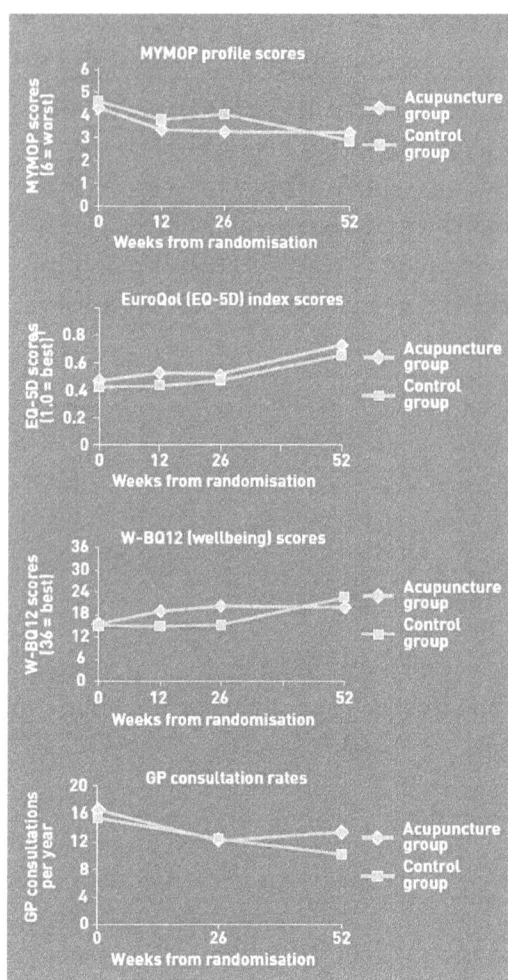

Table 1. Changes in symptoms after Five-element treatment for 12 and 26 weeks and observation up to 52 weeks. [25]

Our Publications

- More Than Acupuncture (book)
- Acupuncture for Emergencies (book)
- Acupuncture Styles in Current Practice (book)
- What We Can Learn from Acupuncture Research in Western Countries (book)
- Does Nora Five-element Acupuncture Depend mostly on Psychological Effect? (book)

Books are available in Amazon.com

References

[1] 龙梅 (译）. 诺娜·弗兰格林 (著).《五行针灸指南》. 中国中医药出版社.
【Long Mei (translator), Nora Flaglen (Author). 《Guide of Five-element Acupuncture》. China Traditional Chinese Medicine Press. Bejing. 2013
】http://pan.baidu.com/share/link?shareid=3777340260&uk=3626297757&adapt=pc&fr=ftw

[2] 饮水斋.北京五行针灸生活群中老师对一次病例的讨论.【Yin Shui Zan. Case Discussion in web group of Five-element acupuncture in Beijing】. http://www.weixindou.com/p/M6298YZS60.html

[3] Wang M. Acupuncture in current practice.
https://www.researchgate.net/publication/314040632_Acupuncture_in_current_practice

[4] Wang M. 针灸不是心理作用 - 西方针刺研究中的缺陷和错误 (2ed).【Acupuncture is not placebo – errors and mistakes in Acupuncture research in Western countries.】http://www.weixindou.com/p/M6298YZS60.html

[5] Moseley JB, O'Malley K, Petersen NJ, Menke TJ, Brody BA, Kuykendall DH, Hollingsworth JC, Ashton CM, Wray NP. A controlled trial of arthroscopic surgery for osteoarthritis of the knee. N Engl J Med, 2002,347(2):81-88

[6] Guyuron B, Reed D, Kriegler JS, Davis J, Pashmini N, Amini S. A placebo-controlled surgical trial of the treatment of migraine headaches. Plast Reconstr Surg. 2009;124:461–468.

[7] Wang M. Placebo effect, sham acupuncture and acupuncture research.
https://www.researchgate.net/publication/311714490_Placebo_effect_sham_acupuncture_and_acupuncture_research

[8] 佟博然. 五行针灸—寻找真实的自我.【Tong Bo-ran. Five-element Acupuncture – seek for true ourselves】.
http://www.360doc.com/content/15/0831/06/11385461_495931735.s

html

9 仙人掌艾灸养生的博客。[转载]血压及脉压差.【Blog of Moxibustion Healthcare by XIanrenzhang. Cited: Blood pressure and pressure difference】.
http://blog.sina.com.cn/s/blog_602b6b950102e8uo.html

10 维基百科.
【Wikipedia】.https://zh.wikipedia.org/wiki/%E9%AB%98%E8% A1%80%E5%A3%93

11 王蓉, 刘妍, 陈瑶, 刘叶, 周密. 艾灸治疗原发性高血压病的探讨. 护理实践与研究 2013 年 10 卷 04 期 33-34 页.【Wang R. Liu Y. Chen Y. Liu Y. Zhou M. Treatment of primary hypertension with moxibustion. Nursing Practice and Research. 2013,10(4):33-34】.

12 孙道霞. 艾灸足三里穴辅助治疗老年高血压的护理要点体会. 中国保健营养 2016 年 26 卷 07 期 250 页.【Sun DX. Experience in the use of moxibusion as complementary treatment and nursing for elderly hypertension】. China Health Care & nutrition. 2016, 26(7): 250

13 刘雅秋.艾灸足三里穴治疗老年高血压患者 135 例临床护理观察.世界最新医学信息文摘(电子版) 2014 年 11 期 244-244,241 页.【Liu YQ. Clinic observation on Moxibustion treatment on Zusanli point for 135 cases of elderly hypertension】. World Latest Medicine Information. 2014, 11: 244, 241.

14 http://www.yusoo.com.tw/mobile.php?dir= Physiognomy&web=five_elements

15 麦玲玲.面相. 五行面相特征与婚配吉凶.【Mai LL. Face future prediction. Characteristics of Five-element face and marry future】.http://blog.sina.com.cn/s/blog_b708a0860102uxlt.html

16 金自在看相—如何辨識你是哪種五行人.【Jin SZ. Face prediction – how to tell which element you are】.
https://www.lnka.tw/html/topic/8911.html

17 雨揚居士.相學五行觀——知人先知面.【Yu Y. (lay Buddhist). Five-element in Face prediction – know the face before knowing the

person】. http://www.epochtimes.com/b5/11/4/11/n3224508.htm

[18] 费秉勋.人相学. 人民中国出版社【Fei BX. Face prediction】.
People's Publishing House of China 1993.5.

[19] 壹读.神奇的「鬼門十三針」療法.【Yi D. Mysterious 'Ghost 13
needle acupuncture'】. https://read01.com/gRx4kG.html

[20] **湖心亭看雪客.**鬼灵附体所致精神病的诊断与治疗方法.【Hu Xin Ting
Kan Xue Ke. The diagnosis and treatment of mental diseases due to
ghost attachment】.
http://blog.sina.com.cn/s/blog_49b5473f0100bhsb.html

[21] 修心微记. 因果病 | 密宗治病、针灸、算命生死、灵附体...【Xiu Xin
Wei Ji. Causal disease. Treatment by Tantra. Acupuncture, Future
prediction, Attached spirit】.
http://m.weixindou.com/p/8C9JAEV249.html

[22] 北京泓道醫學研究院。傳奇針灸---鬼門十三針.【Hong Do Medical
institute, Beijing. Mysterious Acupuncture – Ghost 13 needle acupuncture .
】. https://kknews.cc/health/aj6pj.html

[23] 針灸「十三鬼穴」，您真的了解嗎？【"Ghost 13 needle acupuncture",
do you really understand it？】. https://kknews.cc/health/aopmkj.html

[24] Paterson C, Taylor RS, Griffiths P, Britten N, Rugg S, Bridges J,
McCallum B, Kite G; CACTUS study team. Acupuncture for 'frequent
attenders' with medically unexplained symptoms: a randomised controlled
trial (CACTUS study). Br J Gen Pract. 2011 Jun;61(587):e295-305. doi:
10.3399/bjgp11X572689.

[25] David Colquhoun. Acupuncturists show that acupuncture doesn't
work, but conclude the opposite: journal fails.
http://www.dcscience.net/2011/05/31/acupuncturists-show-that-
acupuncture-doesnt-work-but-conclude-the-opposite-journal-fails/

[26] David Colquhoun (UCL) and Steven Novella. Acupuncture is a
theatrical placebo.
http://www.dcscience.net/2013/05/30/acupuncture-is-a-theatrical-
placebo-the-end-of-a-myth/

www.ingramcontent.com/pod-product-compliance
Lightning Source LLC
Chambersburg PA
CBHW072016230526
45468CB00021B/1627